YOU ARE NOT SELFISH

By
Ameshia Arthur

Copyright © 2025 Ameshia Arthur

All rights reserved.

No part of this publication may be reproduced, distributed, or transmitted in any form or by any means, including photocopying, recording, or other electronic or mechanical methods, without the prior written permission of the author or publisher, except in the case of brief quotations embodied in critical reviews and certain other noncommercial uses permitted by copyright law.

Table of Contents

Introduction 1

Chapter 1: You Are Not Selfish 3

Chapter 2: What Will You Burn For? 6

Chapter 3: Rethinking Your Womanhood 11

Chapter 4: Romance: The Myth of Self-Sacrifice 15

Chapter 5: Selfish vs. Sacrifice 20

Chapter 6: Listen to Her: The Cost of Stress 25

Chapter 7: Ways to Replenish 33

Chapter 8: How Do You Love Yourself? 42

Chapter 9: What Do You Need to Be Healthy? An inventory 46

Chapter 10: Boundaries and Isolation 53

Chapter 11: Then What Is Community? 60

Conclusion: Let's Heal Ourselves with Selfishness 65

Introduction

"We were never meant to survive, not as human beings. And neither were most of you here today, Black or not. The machine will try to grind you into dust, whether or not we speak."
— Audre Lorde, The Cancer Journals

You were never meant to survive.
Not to sustain, not to replenish, not to thrive.
You were meant to be a sacrifice, for family, for community, for commerce.

This world has never needed you to last, only to burn bright enough to light the way for others while turning to ash yourself.

If they believe you were born to be consumed, to warm them with your fire, to illuminate their spaces with your brilliance, is it any wonder they see your survival as selfish?
They never intended for you to rest, to heal, to renew.
They only needed you to reproduce and to teach Black girls that they, too, should go out in a blaze. Disposable. One use.

But what if you refuse?

What if you decide to remain?
To sustain. To flourish. To become wise and whole, connected to a community that does not demand your depletion but instead nourishes your becoming?

If you choose to survive, if you choose yourself, then you are a threat, because a woman who refuses to be consumed cannot be controlled.
And a Black woman who refuses to be sacrificed is the most dangerous of all.

You picked up this book because you hear the call. You feel the misalignment.
Something is off, and girl, it is not you.

I've spent years sitting with women helping them examine themselves in minute detail, trying to fix it.
Their relationships. Their attitudes. Their sadness.
They were being ground down under the weight of *strong*, *good*, and *selfless*.
I know what this costs us.

This book is me talking to myself.
It's my mother talking to me, and us talking to my niece.
It's every conversation I've had with my friends, trying to figure out what is even happening, and how we can fix it.

This book is what I didn't know I was studying for.
And every way, as a therapist, I have walked beside another woman into her healing.

This is my love letter to you.
My wish for our collective survival.

I am a Black woman writing to Black women.
And I am also a woman writing to every other woman, Black or not, who was tricked into thinking the real problem is her.
I welcome all women who've been trained to disappear, defer, or deplete themselves. That lie is over and done with.
We are here to survive together.

You are not broken.
The expectations are.
Your desire to be whole is not selfish, it's sane.

In these pages, you'll find truth-telling, healing, and permission to reclaim your time, your body, your voice, and your peace.
This is not a guide to help you fit the expectation. This is a call to become fully, fearlessly yourself.

In this book, we make a choice to survive. If survival is selfish
Let them call you selfish. Let's show them selfish.

Chapter 1

You Are Not Selfish

"We must learn to live from the inside out."
—bell hooks

What if putting yourself first wasn't selfish? What if it was sacred? For generations, Black women have been told that our power lies in our selflessness. That our strength is proven by how much we can carry. That the more we give, the more we're worth.

We've internalized this story. Carried it in our backs, our bellies, our blood pressure. Made ourselves small, made ourselves useful, made ourselves martyrs. We've called it love. We've called it legacy. We've called it "what Black women do."

But it's not working anymore.

We are exhausted. Not just tired, *depleted*. Giving from empty cups and smiling while we do it. Suppressing our pain to keep the peace. Making everyone else's comfort the measure of our value.

So let me say this clearly:

You are not selfish for wanting to breathe. You are not selfish for having needs.
You are not selfish for choosing yourself.

This book is not an invitation to become cold, detached, or careless. It is an invitation to become *whole*. To examine the lies you've been told about love, labor, womanhood, and worth, and to reclaim your time, your energy, your body, and your joy.

It's a rejection of the binary that says women can either give everything or be selfish. It's a reclamation of your right to be *strategic*, to be *discerning*, to be *well*.

This book is for the caretakers. The overfunctioners.
The ones who hold space for everyone else but feel guilty when they need care, too.

This book is for the eldest daughters. The strong friends.
The mothers, aunties, grandmothers, sisters, play cousins, and community builders.
The ones who were taught that your goodness lies in how much you give, even if it costs you everything.

This book is for you.

Because even though the world may not say it often enough: *your life matters*. Not just what you do for others. Not just your survival. Your *thriving*. Your full expression. Your ability to say "yes" and "no" with clarity and confidence.

We will not heal by accident. We will not rest our way into liberation by waiting for someone else to give us permission.

We have to choose a different way. That starts here.

~Reflection Page~

Chapter 2

What Will You Burn For?

"Tell them about how you are never really a whole person if you remain silent because there is always that one little piece inside of you that wants to be spoken out and if you keep ignoring it it gets madder and madder and hotter and hotter and if you don't speak it out one day it will just up and punch you in the mouth."
— Audre Lorde

Let's start with a question:
What is selfishness? How is it defined? Who gets to define it?

Here's the truth: what's considered "selfish" depends almost entirely on what others expect from you. If you deviate from the role they've assigned, especially if you do so in defense of your health, your joy, or your time, they may call you selfish. Not because you are, but because you've disrupted the arrangement.

So let's name that arrangement.

If the world expects you to create art, and you don't because you'd rather rest, you're selfish. If the world expects you to have and raise children, and you choose not to, you're selfish.
If the world expects you to give until there's nothing left, and you say no, you're selfish.

And if you're a Black woman? That word carries even more weight. Because the expectation placed on you isn't just about giving. It's about giving everything. Your labor. Your wisdom. Your time. Your body. Your brilliance. Your softness. Your silence.

And when you don't?

You're not just called selfish, you're made to feel guilty. Unworthy.

Difficult. Disposable. But here's what I want to offer you today:
If you've survived in a world that expects your self-erasure, you've already been selfish. And I'm proud of you.

Let's keep going.

The Machinery of Expectation

So how does society maintain this dynamic, this extraction, this depletion? It does it slowly. Subtly. Repetitively.
Through media. Through praise and punishment. Through beauty standards and gender roles. And often, through the way we are conditioned to relate to one another as women.

One especially harmful tool is the idea that a woman's value is tied to her youth. This lie creates distance between generations. It paints older women as bitter, outdated, or invisible, just as they're beginning to break free of society's illusions. And it paints younger women as naive or disloyal if they choose to listen to their elders.

This is no accident. It's a design.

Because a community of women who trust each other, who listen to each other, who learn from each other? That's powerful. That's a problem for anyone trying to control us.

So we're encouraged to be isolated, competitive, disconnected. But you and I? We're not falling for it.

Reclaiming the Right to Choose

This book isn't asking you to stop loving people. It's not calling you to selfishness in the way the world defines it, it's calling you to clarity. To intention. To asking yourself *why* before you give.

There are causes worth sacrificing for. Absolutely. There are people, principles, communities, and futures that deserve your energy.

But what if you had a say in what those were? What if you got to choose?

That's the shift.

I'm not telling you to stop showing up. I'm telling you to stop disappearing when you do it.

Adjusting the Dial

You might be at 130%. You're exhausted, aching, but still trying to give more.
What if you gave 65% instead? What if that was enough? What if you were enough?

The goal here isn't to do nothing, it's to stop doing everything. Not because you don't care, but because you do.

Because you want to be here for the long game: To age well.
To witness the fruits of your labor. To laugh.
To rest.
To love.
To pass down stories.
To dance at someone's wedding or graduation or backyard barbecue and know your presence is still medicine.

My Mother

My mother died of cancer. She gave everything.
I don't think she regretted her sacrifices, but I do wish she had known what was being demanded of her. Fully. With all the costs laid out clearly.

I wish she had been told that her rest mattered. That her joy was not optional.
That her energy was not a debt to be collected on until death.

This chapter isn't about blaming her, or you, or any of us. It's about breaking the silence long enough to ask:

Is there another way?

Questions to Guide You

When you're about to give, ask:

- Why am I doing this?
- Who benefits most from this?
- What happens if I don't do it?
- What does it cost me to say yes?
- Am I willing to pay that price today?
- Can I sustain this? And if not, for how long can I keep pretending?
- Could this pace hurt me?
- What is worth living for?
- What is worth dying for?

And most importantly:

Am I allowed to choose?

Because you are.

Not just for yourself.
But for your legacy.
For the women coming after you.

For the ones who could not choose.
And for the ones who didn't know they could choose.

~Reflection Page~

Chapter 3

Rethinking Your Womanhood

"That man over there says that women need to be helped into carriages, and lifted over ditches, and to have the best place everywhere. Nobody ever helps me into carriages, or over mud- puddles, or gives me any best place! And ain't I a woman?...Then that little man in black there, he says women can't have as much rights as men, 'cause Christ wasn't a woman! Where did your Christ come from? Where did your Christ come from? From God and a woman! Man had nothing to do with Him."
—Sojourner Truth

What were you taught it means to be a woman? Your answer will be shaped by your intersections, your culture, your race, your religion, your body, your class. As Sojourner Truth's words highlight, white women were told they were delicate, in need of protection and guidance. Black women were told they weren't women at all. We were positioned as strong, resilient, unbreakable, mules, not maidens.

Though those depictions seem opposite on the surface, they share a dangerous common thread: both are rooted in powerlessness and servitude. Both are designed to benefit men and the systems they uphold.

No one teaches us to question these messages. But that's exactly what we're here to do.

It's time to curate your own definition of womanhood, one that reflects your values, your experiences, your intersecting identities. It's time to look at what's been handed to you, and decide what's worth keeping and what needs to be returned to sender.

We're introduced to womanhood through roles.

From birth, a girl is named "daughter." There's nothing inherently wrong with that, it's often true. But baked into that label is a set of expectations: to care, to serve, to behave.

Take "eldest daughter syndrome," for example. It's not "eldest child syndrome", it's daughter. That tiny distinction reveals a deeper truth: girl children, especially the firstborn, are expected to carry more. More responsibility. More emotional labor. More silence. Less freedom.

And that's just the beginning.

As girls grow, the next set of roles is quickly introduced: bride and mother. We're given baby dolls and toy kitchens. We're praised for being nurturing. We're asked who we're going to marry, long before we even understand the institution of marriage. We're read fairy tales where the happiest ending is the ring, the wedding, the prince.

This isn't about whether you want to be married or have children. This is about how early and how often womanhood is framed as being in service to others. Be his helpmate. Be his peace. Be a good wife. A good mother.

I want to pause here and acknowledge: not all women partner with men, and not all mothers are in traditional family structures. But the script, the archetype of woman-as-caregiver, is rooted in a heteronormative, patriarchal model. It shapes all of us, even if we reject it.

Within that model, a woman is expected to give. To care. To serve.

And if she doesn't become a wife or mother? She's still expected to explain why not. To justify her life. To make her joy, her peace, her freedom, understandable to others. Because womanhood, as defined by society, is synonymous with enthusiastic sacrifice.

I have known beautiful, loving, powerful, single, child-free women. I have been present as person after person asks heartbreaking, rude, and selfish coded questions: Why are you single? What is wrong with you?

You don't want kids? Don't you think that's selfish? Girl, you're getting up there, you better settle down.

As if every woman with a lifestyle that doesn't fit the stereotype chose that life, and did so because she is defective and/or selfish.

We're told women are born to nurture. That we don't need help, we *are* the help. It's time to interrupt that script. And write something new.

~Reflection Page~

Chapter 4

Romance: The Myth of Self-Sacrifice

Healthy love does not require self-abandonment.
—*Nedra Glover Tawwab*

A teenage girl once told me about her heartache. She cared deeply for a boy. She showed her love the way many girls are taught to, by checking in, offering emotional support, listening to him vent about his family and the pressure of sports. Though they were "just friends," she prioritized him, made space for him, and poured herself into his wellbeing. One day, clearly distressed and unable to focus on her own goals, she told me he had started dating someone else.

Heartbroken, she turned to the adults in her life for comfort, and was told, "If you love him, you'll keep trying."

Wait. What?

What the actual hell?

Let's be clear: this advice came from people who loved her. But that's exactly the problem. This wasn't just bad advice, it was a lesson. A coded message: *Your pain doesn't matter. Your needs don't matter. If you're good enough, patient enough, selfless enough… he'll come around.*

As a therapist, I am trained to hold space, to support without judgment, to help people find their own answers. But I couldn't let that moment pass. Because it wasn't just about her, it was about all of us.

This is the myth so many women grow up on: the idea that love is earned through self-sacrifice. That if you are kind enough, calm enough, loyal enough, he will change for you. That being a "good woman" means patiently enduring an emotionally unavailable man until he becomes the partner you deserve.

But let me be clear, as a seasoned, credentialed mental health professional: That is not how humans change.

That's not a love story. It's a blueprint for burnout.
It's not romance. It's codependency dressed up in a pretty dress.

Thankfully, many in the next generation are starting to challenge these old tropes. They're looking more critically at what they're being taught about love. But make no mistake, the myths haven't disappeared. They've just been rebranded. Today, it's still often presented like this:

You? Be perfect. Him? Be broken.
And the test of your worth? Whether he changes for you.

Black women are reminded how rare they get to participate in marriage. How undesirable they are. This story is rehearsed in media, social media, and community discourse. Black women are made to believe that their loyalty through hardship is their only redeeming quality, and the only way we will ultimately be chosen.

We've got to retire this story.

Because here's the truth: people do not change because someone else loved them hard enough. People change when they decide to. When they commit to doing the work. Not because you cooked more meals, listened longer, had more sex, forgave more mistakes, or prayed harder.

So, what is romance, really?

Romance is not martyrdom. It is not endurance. It is not a reward for emotional labor.

It's a mutual experience of care, connection, and accountability. It is not your job to mold someone into their best self by sacrificing your own.

Yes, love can be transformative. But not at the cost of your peace, your energy, or your wholeness.

So what can we do instead? We get selfish.
We get curious.
We ask:

What do I want in a romantic relationship? What do I expect to give? What beliefs about love am I ready to release?

Here's a foundational concept I'll offer you:
Discernment is a gift. Use it early.

Stop hoping that a problematic partner will "bloom" into someone else just because you're beautiful, accomplished, or loyal enough to inspire him. Most people's core personality traits remain relatively stable in adulthood. According to the research, personality is not fixed, but neither is it easily changed.

"The literature on rank-order stability provides strong evidence that individual differences in personality traits are stable across many decades... leaving room for personality trait change throughout the lifespan."
—Sage Journals, 2023

Change is possible. I believe in it, I'm a therapist!
But change that's real and sustainable is never about your worthiness or

your sacrifice. So how do we reclaim romance? How do we apply

selfishness here?

Start by choosing you, and being honest about what you want, what you're willing to give, and what you are no longer available for. Be honest about the ways you've been trained to see love as a reward for labor, and begin dismantling that conditioning.

Romantic partnership doesn't require sameness, but it should involve *mutual benefit*. I like the image of a mutualistic symbiotic relationship, a long-term connection between two distinct beings where both thrive. That's what you deserve. Not to be drained. Not to be used. Not to be waiting for someone else's potential to finally show up.

So here's the invitation:
Pour into love, yes. But pour into yourself, too. Give, but take, receive, expect.
And believe that romance, real romance, begins with self-regard, not self-abandonment.

The world is yours now.
What a beautiful, selfish question to ask: How can I love and still keep more for me?

~Reflection Page~

Chapter 5

Selfish vs. Sacrifice

"Anyone interested in making change in the world also has to learn how to take care of herself."
—*Angela Davis*

Let's be clear:
Not helping when you can is the harmful selfish.
Asking for more and contributing nothing is harmful selfish. Refusing to support shared goals is harmful selfish.
But being tired? Being human? That's not harmful or selfish. That's honest.

Sometimes, it feels easier to be used.
We're rewarded for being useful. Applauded for our sacrifice. Spoken of fondly if we've "given it all." There's approval in that, and it can feel good.

This is one way women are trained into people-pleasing. Women are conditioned to measure our worth by how much we give away. Black women are measured by how much suffering we can endure in our roles as strong Black women, pillars of the family, or the ride-or-die in a partnership.

The training runs deep. And even once we become aware of it, it's hard to break. After all, if pleasing others feels good and earns praise, what's the harm?

Here's the harm:
"Use me up" leaves us used up.
And used up is an unhealthy, unfulfilled husk.

The Cost of Constant Sacrifice

Stress is part of life. We're not trying to eliminate it, we're trying to balance it. One helpful framework for this is the Yerkes-Dodson Law, which shows that moderate stress supports optimal performance, but too much leads to burnout. On the other end, too little stress leads to stagnation.

Think of a bell curve. On the far left: under-functioning, isolation, and avoidance. On the far right: strain, depletion, and martyrdom. Right in the middle? That's where our contributions lead to growth, not collapse.

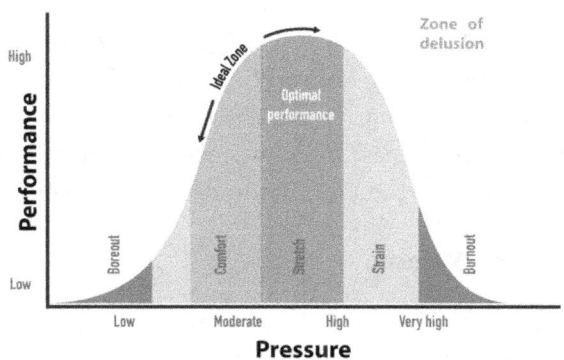

Martyrs live on the far right of that curve. One definition of martyr? A constant sufferer.

They give until there's nothing left, and often feel bitter, tired, and unseen. Many women, especially those raised to be caretakers, say:
"I have to."
"If I don't, who will?"
"If I love you, I give it all."

But that logic is killing us.
Giving it all isn't the only way to show love. And burnout isn't a badge of honor.

Let's reframe what it means to give. Let's experiment with selfishness, not as neglect, but as self-protection. Let's move from burnout to balance.

From Burnout to Balance: Meet Marion

Marion is in her thirties. She has a full life, friends, a partner, aging parents, and a beloved dog. She works over forty hours a week and volunteers for an animal rights organization she cares deeply about. She supports her parents financially, gives them rides to appointments, shows up for her friends' events, and fosters two puppies in addition to caring for her elderly dog. She manages Type 1 diabetes, takes pride in being an emotional rock for her partner, and is known as someone everyone can count on.

And yet, Marion feels exhausted. Her body is tired, her health is declining, and despite being constantly surrounded by people, she often feels lonely. She rarely shares her own struggles because she doesn't want to burden anyone. She wants to exercise but never has the time. She's doing everything "right", but she's running on empty.

Now, meet **Selfish Marion**.

Selfish Marion still works full-time, but she no longer takes on voluntary overtime. She's narrowed her volunteer efforts to just two projects a year, causes she's deeply passionate about. She helps her parents within a sustainable budget and gives rides one Saturday a month and has let her siblings know more support may be needed. This has make time with her parents less stressful and more meaningful.

She attends her closest friends' milestone events and coordinates hangouts that fit into her schedule. She's paused fostering new dogs to focus on caring for her elderly pup in his final years. She's enrolled in a diabetes support program and is learning to manage her health more effectively.

She still takes pride in being an emotional safe space for her partner, but now allows herself to receive care, too. She reaches out to friends, family, or a therapist when she's having a hard day. Her sleep is improving, her health is stabilizing, and she's begun to exercise, sometimes. And when she doesn't, she offers herself compassion instead of shame.

The difference?
Marion didn't become selfish at the expense of others. She became selfish in service of alignment.
She became strategic with her time, energy, and love.
She still contributes, but now in ways that support her well-being, so her community can experience a fuller, healthier Marion for years to come. Small changes. Big impact.

Journal Prompts: What About You?

What does being "selfish" stir up in me?
Where am I operating in burnout instead of balance? Who am I trying to prove myself to by over-giving?
What do I need to say no to, even if it disappoints someone?
Who do I fear will stop loving or respecting me if I stop over-giving?
What would a life of sustainable contribution look like for me?

Let's not wait until we're used up.
Let's not call sacrifice love when it's actually depletion. Let's be selfish, like Marion.
Not in neglect, but in alignment. Let's be in balance.

~Reflection Page~

Chapter 6

Listen to Her: The Cost of Stress

"That stress will kill you."
— *Brigitte Gabriel*

The Truth We Already Knew

I knew that stress was dangerous before I even knew what it was. Long before grad school, licensure, or reading a single research paper, I knew it with the gut certainty of a child repeating her mother: *stress will kill you.*

That wisdom was passed down to me, not from a textbook, but from a woman with generational knowledge, earned through life, loss, and survival. My mother didn't need peer-reviewed studies to understand the cost of carrying too much, for too long. But now, science agrees: chronic stress is not just emotionally exhausting, it's biologically dangerous.

This chapter, like this book, is a call to be selfish in the most radical way: to care for yourself like your life depends on it, because it does. To stop waiting for collapse to justify rest. To stop needing someone else's permission to pay attention to your own body.

What Stress Really Is

Before we go deeper, let's ground ourselves in the basics:

- **Stress:** A state of mental or emotional tension caused by difficult situations.

- **Chronic stress:** When stress becomes long-term, lasting weeks or months.

- **Stress response:** The body's physiological reaction, your heart rate rises, your muscles tense, cortisol floods your system. This response was designed for short bursts of danger. But when it's activated over and over, day after day, it becomes toxic.

Stress can be internal or external. It can come from your environment, your relationships, your finances, or your thoughts. Some stressors are within your control. Many are not. Most lie somewhere in between.

What *is* firmly in your control is your response. That's what this chapter is about: identifying what's within your reach, and reclaiming your power to respond intentionally, without blame, without shame, and with full awareness of the stakes.

This is not a call for individual bootstrapping in the face of systemic injustice. Yes, stress is worsened by racism, poverty, homophobia, misogyny, and all the ways institutions grind people down. That context matters.

But understanding the impact of chronic stress on your health is not about fault. It's about survival. And choosing to *be selfish enough to survive.*

This Isn't Just in Your Head

Medical and psychological communities have long established what the wisdom keepers in our communities already knew: chronic stress wreaks havoc on the body. Poverty, trauma, food insecurity, housing instability, violence, and isolation all function as long-term stressors. And they don't just exhaust you emotionally, they cause real, measurable damage.

Chronic stress touches *every* system in the body. Studies show that people living or working in high-stress environments are more likely to develop disease. And women, especially Black women, are bearing the brunt.

Research Roundup

Stress and Autoimmune Disease

- Up to 80% of patients with autoimmune diseases reported serious emotional stress before symptoms began.
  Source: Stojanovich & Marisavljevich, 2008

- A meta-analysis of over 3,200 patients confirmed that people with autoimmune diseases were significantly more likely to have experienced major life stressors before illness onset.
  Source: Porcelli et al., 2020

- Chronic stress may not just trigger, but worsen the progression of conditions like lupus, rheumatoid arthritis, multiple sclerosis, and scleroderma, particularly in women.
  Source: Yaribeygi et al., 2017

Black Women, Suppressed Emotion, and Heart Disease

- Black women who frequently suppress their anger are 70% more likely to develop carotid artery plaque, a major risk factor for heart attacks and strokes.
  Source: University of Pittsburgh study, cited in Atlanta Tribune, 2024

- Self-silencing, or consistently holding in thoughts and feelings to keep peace, has been linked to IBS, chronic fatigue, and even cancer in women.

- *Source: Atlanta Tribune, 2024, "Silent Rage Is a Hidden Health Crisis Among Women of Color"*

The Full-Body Toll of Stress

Stress doesn't just affect the mind, it impacts every major system:

- **Cardiovascular:** High blood pressure, heart attacks, and "broken heart syndrome"

- **Gastrointestinal:** Acid reflux, IBS, gastritis

- **Immune:** Weakened immune response, frequent illness

- **Endocrine:** Blood sugar imbalances, worsened diabetes

- **Neurological:** Headaches, memory problems, anxiety

- **Musculoskeletal:** Tension, jaw clenching, muscle pain

- **Behavioral:** Overeating, substance use, social withdrawal
  Sources: Mayo Clinic Staff, 2024; Yaribeygi et al., 2017; APA 2024

When Silence Hurts

Let's talk specifically about one stressor that many women carry silently: self-silencing.

Self-silencing is a relational survival strategy. It is the learned practice of suppressing your voice, your needs, and your boundaries to maintain peace, preserve relationships, or avoid punishment. Many of us learned it young, praised for being "mature," "good," "strong," or "easygoing" while swallowing our pain whole.

Over time, this suppression becomes automatic, unconscious, and devastating.

Medical research now confirms that self-silencing isn't just a psychological hazard; it's a physical one. Studies link it to:

- Autoimmune diseases

- Irritable bowel syndrome

- Chronic fatigue syndrome

- HIV progression
- Cardiovascular disease
- Premature death

In one study out of the University of Pittsburgh, women of color who strongly agreed with statements like "I rarely express my anger to those close to me" were 70% more likely to experience carotid artery plaque, an indicator of higher risk for heart attacks and strokes.

Another long-term study found that women who silenced themselves during arguments with their spouses were four times more likely to die prematurely than those who spoke up. *Four times.*

This is not about attitude. This is about survival.
Silence has a cost, and for many women, that cost is the body. Be selfish. Speak up.

Have You Normalized Stress?

It sounds like a simple question. But many women don't know how to answer it honestly. We've been conditioned to dismiss our pain, downplay our fatigue, and keep going. So we adapt to dysfunction until dysfunction becomes our baseline. We forget what it feels like to be calm.

Here's a reality check:

- Do you have chronic fatigue, brain fog, or frequent colds?
- Do you carry unexplained aches or digestive issues?
- Do you often feel numb, irritable, or emotionally detached?
- When was your last physical exam or blood work?
- Do you trust your own perception of your needs?

If you're unsure, ask a friend you trust. Sometimes the people who love us can name what we've normalized. Healing happens in community. Let someone reflect you back to yourself.

Start Small, Stay Alive

The goal isn't to eliminate all stress. The goal is to stop letting it accumulate unexamined. To be selfish enough to notice, to intervene, and to survive.

Here are some small but powerful places to begin:

- **Body scan meditation:** A grounding practice to help you check in without judgment. (Many free recordings available online.)

- **Movement:** Stretching, walking, dancing, anything that gets energy moving.

- **Breathwork:** Deep, intentional breathing signals your nervous system that you are safe.

- **Sleep and hydration:** These basics aren't luxuries. They're resilience tools.

- **Check-ins:** Ask yourself throughout the day, *What am I feeling? What do I need?*

These are ways to show your body you're listening. To lessen stress. To repair self-trust.

Listen to Her

You don't need to wait for a crisis to start caring for yourself.

Be selfish.

Stop performing peace

it's making you sick.

Your stress is real. Your voice is honest.

Your body is telling the truth. Listen to her.

~Reflection Page~

Chapter 7

Ways to Replenish

"As much as creating is important and fulfilling, remember that rest is a kind of devotion too."
—*Well-Read Black Girl, 2025*

Are you tired of hearing about self-care? Me too, girl. You're doing your best, and still, when someone brings up self-care, it feels like just another thing to do. Another area where you're not measuring up. I get it.

This journey can feel so guilt-ridden. Trying to be selfish, balanced, and healthy can feel like just learning all the things we're not doing right. But that's not the intention of this chapter.

Yes, we're going to talk about being selfish enough to replenish yourself regularly. But I'm not here to tell you what you *should* be doing. I'm here to remind you that you are worthy of care.

I'm offering ideas, not demands. Invitations, not obligations. So park the guilt. Let go of the judgment. Come with curiosity.
Look for one thing that feels good. One small way to move toward wholeness. One moment to be selfish enough to care for *you*.

When I talk with clients about self-care, I offer them a simple definition:

Self-care is an act of care that makes you feel better during or after, and

you don't regret it later. That's it.
Not what someone else says should feel good.
Not something that makes you look like you've got your life together.
Not something you squeeze in once a year to reset from burnout.
Something that feels like care, in the moment or soon after, and doesn't

leave you drained, ashamed, or depleted later.

That definition is powerful in its simplicity, but there's more.

Self-care is the ongoing practice of doing things that improve your well-being or quality of life, especially before things fall apart.

Ideally, self-care helps prevent mental and physical overwhelm. It creates room for you to exhale and stay connected to yourself.

That longer definition matters because self-care isn't a destination, it's a rhythm. A practice. Like tending a garden or brushing your teeth. If we forget that, we might feel like we're doing it wrong just because we have to keep doing it.

But care isn't something you complete, it's something you return to.

Think of how we maintain everything else we value, our homes, our cars, our relationships. Why should our well-being be the exception?

Meet Magda

Magda is a composite of many women I've partnered with on the road to balance, healing, and selfishness.

She came to therapy unsure what was wrong, just that something was. She described feeling deeply depressed about going to work, but said she didn't feel much better at home. She believed she was doing everything wrong and had been "lazy lately."

When I asked Magda to walk me through a typical day, here's what she shared:
She wakes at 5 a.m. to work a bit before her kids get up. Then she wakes her three small children, gets them ready for school, and drops them off. From there, she heads straight to work and puts in six hours. After work, she picks up the kids, makes dinner, helps with homework, handles bedtime, and often squeezes in a bit more work before she passes out.

She's kept this pace for eight years.

When I asked about rest, Magda laughed: "When?"

When we began discussing self-care, she insisted it was impossible to fit into her life. And honestly? Her concern made sense. Her pace wasn't sustainable, but like many women, she had been surviving, not replenishing.

Together, we explored what could shift. Not everything. Just *something*.

We came up with a plan: a regular playdate with a longtime friend. While the kids were away, Magda wasn't allowed to work. She had to do something that felt good to her body. The playdate would happen twice a month, and so would her rest.

Even though they felt small, Magda noticed something: the week before her self-care day, she felt a lift just from having something to look forward to. The week of, she had more patience and energy.

Now, she's excited. She's dreaming. She's discovering what else might replenish her. Magda, a selfish lady after our own hearts.

Magda found her entry point. It wasn't extravagant, it was enough. And that's the lesson: replenishment starts small, but it matters deeply.

So let's talk about what care might look like for *you*.

The Categories of Care

To better understand your needs, self-care can be thought of in categories:

- **Physical** – walking, dancing, stretching, increasing healthy foods
- **Mental** – going to therapy, journaling, seeking knowledge

- **Emotional** – feeling your feelings on purpose, speaking kindly to yourself, allowing yourself to cry

- **Spiritual** – prayer, meditation, going to places of worship

- **Overall well-being** – laughing, being in community, napping

Some activities support multiple areas, while others are more targeted. Neither is better or worse, but it can be helpful to notice when your care is lopsided.

For example, you may be a gym girly, hitting the gym five days a week, and still feel drained. That could be because your physical self-care is dialed in, but another area, like emotional or spiritual care, needs tending.

Sometimes we confuse discipline with care. But discipline doesn't always fill the emotional, mental, or spiritual cups. That's why your self-care may be "working" physically, but still feel incomplete.

This is not a call to perfection. This is a call to reflection.

Self-Care Is Not a Luxury

Self-care has been deeply commodified. It's been packaged, branded, and sold to us as something that must be earned, or bought. Those with less disposable income are made to feel like they're doing a bad job at healing.

If you can't justify or afford a gym membership, spa day, meditation retreat, or mental health vacation, the world may try to convince you that you're failing.

Let me be clear: That is classist. That is harmful. And that is a lie.

Our people have always found ways to care for ourselves and each other. The problem isn't that we've failed at care, it's that many of us have been cut off from the community rhythms and cultural practices that once made that care organic.

Community Is a Form of Care

Another crucial form of self-care? Asking for and accepting help.

Not everything has to be done alone. You are not a solitary, self-sustaining system. And you were never meant to be.

Women are often expected to over extend themselves. The myth of the "strong Black woman" doubles down on deprivation and has been weaponized. What once could have meant resilient and powerful has been twisted into: "She doesn't need help. She can handle it."

This narrative isn't a compliment, it's an excuse for lack of support. It shifts blame from systems to individuals, and it creates conditions for exhaustion and burnout.

But legacy-building, child-rearing, healing, and long-term wellness are meant to be achieved with many hands.

Let's reclaim our right to community and connection in the process of care. When considering what you should do yourself and what you might delegate or ask help with, ask:

- What is in my power?

- What is in my capacity, considering my priorities, time, and resources?

- What communities do I contribute to that I might also ask for help in?

- What can I ask for help with?

Because the ultimate goal isn't just self.
The ultimate goal is care, for yourself, and for your people.

Quick Reflection: Are You Replenishing or Just Performing?

Ask yourself:

- What kind of care do I tend to overdo?
- What kind of care do I often neglect?
- Who helps me feel cared for, and do I let them?

No-Cost, Soulful Self-Care

Let's strip self-care of the luxury marketing and return it to something simple, nourishing, and yours. These are replenishment ideas, ways to pour into yourself without needing a credit card or a weekend away. Do what feels good now. Come back later for something new.

- Journaling
- Tapping (Emotional Freedom Technique)
- Consensual sex, with yourself or a trusted partner
- Doing your hair
- Self-acupressure
- Foot soak
- Face steam
- Listening to music
- Walking in nature
- Breathing intentionally

- Hugging someone for a long time
- Cuddling with a pet, or wrapping yourself in a soft blanket
- Praying
- Meditating
- Sitting in the dark or by candlelight for a sensory break
- Dancing
- Drawing or painting
- Giving yourself henna
- Coloring
- Crossword, sudoku, word search
- Knitting, crocheting, or crafting
- Gardening
- Biking
- Cooking or baking something comforting
- Getting your heart rate up
- Taking a nap
- Smelling something you love (lavender, citrus, incense, a fresh orange)
- Talking to someone who makes you feel good
- Asking for help

This list is not a prescription. It's a buffet. Take what nourishes you. Leave the rest.

Your replenishment doesn't have to look like anyone else's. It just has

to work for you. Care is not selfish. Care is essential.
And you are worth the investment.

This is not about becoming perfect at care.
It's about becoming selfish enough to stay soft. To stay alive.
To stay you.

~*Reflection Page*~

Chapter 8

How Do You Love Yourself?

"You yourself, as much as anybody in the entire universe, deserve your love and affection."
— Buddha

You're reading this book because you are already brimming with love. You give and give. You pour into others on a regular basis. You likely love hard, loyally and fiercely. But when it comes to loving yourself? So many women like you quietly confess, *I don't even know how to love myself.*

Maybe no one taught you how. Maybe you're simply out of practice.

Maybe when you have tried in the past you were called selfish. Lets lean into selfishness again.

Whatever the reason, take a breath. You're not broken, and you're not alone. We just need a place to start.

Think of someone you've loved fiercely. Think about how you treated them. The way you checked in on them, anticipated their needs, showed up when they were hurting. Remember the joy you felt when you could ease their pain or make them smile.

Now, cut and paste.
This is the kind of love we're going to begin practicing for *you*.

The tenderness.
The fierce protectiveness. The patience.
The presence.
That same love, turned inward.

Those kind words you speak to the people you love? Offer them to yourself. The way you sit beside someone through their dark moments, without judgment or shame? Offer that same loyalty to yourself.

Here's one way to start:
Find a photo of yourself as a child. If you don't have one, bring up the clearest mental image you can. This is the version of you we begin with. Look at her. See her. Hold her in your heart.

If you send good morning texts to others, send one to her too. Each time you offer care to someone else, imagine yourself multiplying that care and pouring it right back into her. This is your beginning. Treat her with the same kindness you offer so freely to others. Over time, as you reconnect with her, you'll learn what care she specifically needs, and how to give it.

This is slow work. Intimate work. But it is *life work*.
Self-love isn't built through spa days and vacations. It's built in the ordinary moments, through attention, consistency, and care.

And like any relationship, it doesn't need to be perfect. It just needs to be responsive. And evolving.

Now, be prepared for something tender and real: resistance.
You may feel uncomfortable. You may feel undeserving. That doesn't mean you're doing it wrong. That means you're finally doing it. That means you're brushing up against old stories that told you love had to be earned. And harsh and wrong judgements that called you selfish for saving some energy kind words and forgiveness for yourself.

This is important so don't miss it:

You are worthy of love. Not because of what you do, or how well you perform. You are worthy because you exist. Period.

You don't need to fully believe this to begin. Start the practice. The belief will follow.

And if you take only one thing from this chapter, let it be this:

Loving yourself as a verb, daily, imperfectly, and on purpose, is what makes every other kind of love possible.

~Reflection Page~

Chapter 9

What Do You Need to Be Healthy? An inventory

You are your best thing.
—*Toni Morrison*

When was the last time you checked in with yourself? When I work with women, often Black women, in my practice, this is a question they haven't asked themselves in years, if ever. Because "woman as martyr" and "woman as caregiver" are such normalized expectations, many have no external indicators that they're overextending themselves. And we have been carefully taught to ignore internal indicators. A woman's self-neglect doesn't just go unnoticed it is encouraged and praised.

So the first step toward health and healing is a rebellious one:
You have to do something you were told is selfish.
You have to check on *you*. Since many women will be new to this we will first discuss it and then there will be guided prompts to help you try it. First ask
Am I okay?

But let's go further. For caregivers, fixers, and women socialized to always be "on," the knee-jerk answer is: *Yes, I'm okay. I got it.*
So let's use our skills as caregivers and fixers to pour some care upon ourselves

In this exercise, we will check in on ourselves the way we would check on a small child or a beloved pet.

Start with your physical needs:

- Am I hungry?

- Am I thirsty?

- Is my body uncomfortable or in pain?

Then, check in on the non-physical aspects of being "okay":

- Am I fulfilled?

- Am I bored?

- Am I lonely?

- Am I experiencing any emotional discomfort?

Each of these questions can be asked out loud, talking to yourself in the mirror, or even to a photo of yourself.
Pause at least 5 seconds before answering to give yourself space to override the automatic answers you were taught.
Alternatively, you can write your answers. Writing gives you the reflective space to be as honest as possible. Whichever way you choose, this is the beginning of a new habit, a habit of selfishness.

Check in with yourself like you would with your child or your best friend. That is to say: check in regularly, thoroughly, and with compassion.

So what do you do when you get an answer? What if you discover that you're *not* okay?

That's wonderful.
Not wonderful that you're not okay, but wonderful that you've discovered something about yourself.
That information empowers you. You now know something you didn't know before. That is a win.

Some answers will be straightforward. Maybe you realize you've spent all day running around, and you're hungry because you forgot to eat. Now you feed yourself. And not later, now.

Don't say: *I'll eat once I finish this report... or once I call so-and-so back... or once the kids are settled.*
No. Feed yourself as if you're caring for your favorite person. Prioritize yourself, unapologetically.
Be selfish.

Other discoveries might not be so simple.

What if you realize you're not okay, and in fact, you've been feeling lonely most of the time? That's a different kind of need. It might take time, reflection, and support to address. Support can come from loved ones, a therapist, a psychiatrist, or even all of the above. All of these options are valid and okay. It's a smart and brave move to access the help you need. The point here isn't quick fixes. The point is building a habit, one that helps you consistently check in, gain insight, and slowly prioritize making your life better. This work is cumulative.

Many of us will feel guilty for taking so much time to check in. We'll hear the voices of responsibility, of obligation, of everyone else's needs shouting in our heads.

You can tolerate that discomfort.
You *can* be selfish enough to take care of yourself. And I guarantee: it will be worth it.

On the following pages you will find some guided check in prompts. This is not homework. It's help.

Use what serves you, skip what doesn't. This is your time.

Guided Self-Check-In: What Do You Need?
This is your moment. This is not about fixing everything right now. It's about listening to yourself with curiosity, honesty, and compassion.

Step 1: Set the Space

- Find a quiet place where you won't be interrupted.

- You may want a mirror, journal, or simply a few minutes alone with your thoughts.

- Take 3 slow, deep breaths. Release your shoulders. Release your jaw.

Step 2: Check Your Physical Needs

Say the following questions out loud or write your answers down. Pause at least 5 seconds after each one.

- Am I hungry?

- Am I thirsty?

- Is my body uncomfortable or in pain?

- Do I need to stretch, move, or rest?

Prompt: What is one small action I can take in the next 30 minutes to meet one of these needs?

Step 3: Check Your Emotional Needs

Ask these questions slowly and with gentleness:

- Am I feeling fulfilled?

- Am I bored?

- Am I lonely?

- Am I feeling emotionally uncomfortable, anxious, sad, angry, or overwhelmed?

Prompt:
What emotion is asking to be acknowledged right now? What is one kind thing I can say to myself in this moment?

Step 4: Shift Into Self-Compassion

Pretend you are speaking to your younger self if at all possible get a picture of school aged you for this exercise

What would you tell them if they were feeling how you feel now?

- What tone of voice would you use?

Prompt:
Write a short note to yourself using that same tone.
Example: *"I know you're tired. It's okay to rest. You deserve the same care you give to everyone else."*

Step 5: Commit to One Act of Care

Choose one small, immediate action to support yourself today. And remember self care is whatever makes you feel good and or better and you do not regret it later. Below is a list of options but let your own joy guide you

- Dance

- Sing full volume

- Say no to something

- Laugh with someone you love

- Take a quiet moment for yourself even if you don't have time

- Eat a meal you enjoy and enjoy it

- Ask a safe person for help

Your relationship with yourself is the most important one you'll ever have. It deserves your time and effort.
Like any relationship, it needs care. You have to spend time together.
Listen deeply.
Create understanding. And pour into it regularly.

When you nurture your relationship with self, you build self-trust, confidence, emotional intelligence, and the ability to regulate your emotions.
When you neglect it, you create space for distrust, disconnection, and dysfunction. Choose wisely.

~Reflection Page~

Chapter 10

Boundaries and Isolation

"Boundaries are the distance at which I can love you and me simultaneously."
— *Prentis Hemphill*

We are here to be what we have been accused of: selfish. We are not here to accidentally isolate ourselves by misunderstanding the process and purpose of healthy boundaries.

What Are Boundaries?

Boundaries are stated expectations about how you will be treated. They communicate what you are and are not comfortable with. Expectations must be *communicated* and *enforced* in order to qualify as a boundary.

Too Much of a Good Thing

Porous boundaries are ill-defined. They shift with little rhyme or reason and can lead to enmeshment, oversharing, people-pleasing, and burnout.

Rigid boundaries are "my way or the highway" types. They're not flexible or self-aware. Rigid boundaries often come from fear or trauma. These can lead to avoidance and emotional isolation.

Healthy boundaries create safe environments to explore connection. They do not compromise your values. They grow as self-awareness grows. They are flexible and clear. People with healthy boundaries also practice healthy communication.

Begin with the End in Mind

This is your guiding principle.

We hear a lot about boundaries today. We hear about going no contact, standing on business, keeping your circle small, moving in silence, and protecting your peace. These are powerful ideas, but they're repeated so often they've lost their context.

That context is *the life you are building.*

Personal boundaries are the limits and rules we set for ourselves within relationships. They are not ultimatums. They are not weapons. They are not about controlling others.

Boundaries are a *roadmap* for your own behavior. They're about what you will or will not participate in.

Clarify, Communicate, Enforce

A healthy boundary has three steps: it is clarified to self, communicated to others, and enforced if needed. Skip any step, and you're likely doing something other than setting a boundary.

So how do you clarify what your boundaries are?

You start by checking in with yourself. Learn what you need in your relationships to be the healthiest version of you. Some needs, you'll meet yourself. Some, you can ask others to meet. That difference matters.

For example, if a person you're close to asks for space during a disagreement and that request makes you extremely anxious, the work here is *not* about changing them. It's about soothing yourself. Why? Because asking for space can be a healthy and reasonable request. If your nervous system can't tolerate it, that's your work.

Another example: if you become anxious when someone yells during a disagreement, that *is* a place for a boundary. In a calm moment, you can say, "When you yell, I feel anxious. Will you speak to me calmly, at a normal volume?"

If they continue yelling, enforcement is not about asking again, escalating the argument, or trying to change them. Enforcement means removing access to you. You leave the room, hang up the phone, or step away.

Boundaries are not sound bites. They're more complex than we're led to believe.

Not All-or-Nothing

Here's a clip from an article about boundaries: *"Sometimes, no matter how hard you've tried to communicate your boundaries, someone may break them anyway. In that case, know that you're allowed to cut off contact with that person."*

This is the kind of statement that makes boundaries seem black and white, all or nothing, and that's just not real life.

Sure, if an acquaintance crosses your boundary, cutting contact might make sense. But what if it's your parent? Your spouse? Your supervisor?

If you tell your family you don't want to be in the group text and your aunt loops you in anyway, does that mean go no contact? Not necessarily. Maybe you silence the thread, leave it, ignore it, or block it. All are valid forms of enforcement.

If your workplace schedules a 5 PM meeting after you've set the boundary that your workday ends at 5, do you quit? Maybe. But maybe you don't go, maybe you reschedule, maybe you take PTO. Those are all options too.

Boundaries don't require abuse to justify them, but different relationships require different enforcement strategies. That flexibility keeps us from becoming so rigid we end up isolated.

Zoom out. What are you building? What's actually within your control?

Culture and Boundaries

Boundaries take on a different meaning when taking your culture into consideration. Many therapy tools I've discussed in this book are still considered "white people stuff" to communities of color.

And I get it.

Many Black, Mexican, Indian, Tongan, and other nonwhite families live in cultures where collective survival takes priority. In those settings, boundaries may not have had a place in the family's survival story.

If you grew up in a multigenerational household, shared clothes with siblings, had your pay automatically expected to go to household expenses, or watched younger siblings or cousins while their parents worked, you know there wasn't much space for personal boundaries.

And let's be honest: that sacrifice has built strong, supportive, and financially stable families. The strategy works.

But that's also why beginning with the end in mind is so important.

If your family's elevation is a shared priority, maybe your boundaries don't include saying no to everything. Maybe you're still cooking and babysitting, but you set boundaries around time or tone. "I can babysit any day but Sunday." "I will contribute financially, but I'm also saving a portion for my first car."

Your boundaries are your own. They don't have to look like anyone else's.

Build Something Worth Living In

Boundaries are about knowing yourself, your values, your priorities, and your needs. They help you decide: is this my work? Or is this something I need to communicate or choose new people for?

With each boundary you build, you are creating the emotional home you live in. It can be a fortress, a prison, or a dream home.

Healthy boundaries help you build that dream home: based on self-knowledge, communication, and evolution. Notice if your boundaries are keeping everyone out. That's not protection, that's isolation.

That doesn't mean you owe anyone access. But it does mean being honest with yourself: are you hiding behind boundaries because it's easier than being vulnerable?

Healthy boundaries will never leave you without community. Your community may change, but real boundaries leave you surrounded by truth and connection.

Boundaries are not about opting out of relationship. They are how you *navigate* relationship.

Feel It All

It can be hard to say what you need. People will push back, especially those who benefited from your porous boundaries.

That pushback might hurt. The grief of losing a relationship, even an unhealthy one, is real. Let yourself feel it.

And then, come back to your purpose:

Be selfish.

Be selfish enough to survive.

Be selfish and brave enough to let go of what harms you. Be selfish enough to allow new, healthier connections in.

This is not about instant gratification. This is not people-pleasing. This is about building a life that sustains you and lets you thrive. Use the prompts below to reflect on what you need, what you're protecting, and what kind of life you're building with every "yes" and every "no."

Journal Prompts

- What boundaries do you currently have?

- Are they healthy?

- Have you communicated them?

- Can they be enforced?

- Which of my boundaries feel empowering, and which ones might be rooted in fear or past hurt?

- How do I typically respond when someone crosses a boundary I've set?

- Where in my life do I feel most drained? Is a boundary needed there?

- In what relationships do I feel safe enough to be flexible with my boundaries, and where do I need to be firmer?

- How do my cultural background and family values shape how I view and set boundaries?

- What's one boundary I want to set this month, and what will enforcement look like if it's crossed?

~Reflection Page~

Chapter 11

Then What Is Community?

"The revolution will come in love. It will come in connection. It will come in community."
— *Adrienne Maree Brown*

I'm a licensed clinical social worker. A therapist trained in California, shaped by the DSM, and regulated by the California Board of Behavioral Sciences. I say this so you understand: I've been deeply immersed in the traditional, Western model of mental health. But I also carry an intersectional identity and lived experience that compel me to question it.

Western therapy is rooted in individualistic, patriarchal values. In these systems, the individual's needs, goals, and independence are paramount. Personal achievement and self-reliance are celebrated. Directness is valued. Uniqueness is a virtue.

But in communal cultures, the collective is at the center. Shared values, mutual responsibility, interconnection. Belonging isn't just desired, it's the fabric that keeps the community intact. The question is not "Who am I?" but "Who are we, together?" And though no culture is perfect, I've seen firsthand how communal frameworks have supported strong, healthy individuals, and thriving communities.

We are not putting any models of being on a pedestal. Some of us have been most harmed *inside* of community, by family, religious groups, or movements. Keep your critical thinking sharp, whether you're navigating individual or communal cultures. That's how you'll understand the pros and cons. And with that clarity, you're better equipped to make the best decisions for *you*. Community doesn't always mean returning to the same people. Sometimes it means creating something new, rooted in mutual care and accountability.

What happens when we bring communal values into individualistic spaces? We get burned.

We give and give, expecting reciprocity, shared care, a return on love. Instead, we're left depleted. Meanwhile, those who operate from an individualist lens often walk away enriched, proud of their self-sufficiency, and completely unaware of the imbalance.

A History of Misunderstanding

Take the term *"Indian giver."* It came from a deep misunderstanding of Native American gift- giving practices. For many Indigenous communities gifts were part of a non-verbal, mutual exchange. Resources circulated to serve the whole, not hoard for the individual.

European settlers, steeped in individualism, misunderstood this. They thought a gift was something you gave away, never to ask about again. So when reciprocity was expected, they saw it as a betrayal. Hence, the offensive term.

The result? Indigenous people were painted as untrustworthy. The settlers were enriched. A communal practice was distorted by an individualistic lens, and the community who practiced it paid the price.

We're still living this dynamic today.

That's why it's essential to know your values, and the values of the spaces you enter. If you don't, you risk depletion, misinterpretation, and harm.

The Individualism Trap

Western therapy steeped in individualistic values doesn't just strain communal values, it has the potential to harm. But for women, especially those with intersectional identities, the damage may run deep.

Women have long carried the communal role: caregivers, organizers, emotional anchors. I hope you see by now this book isn't asking you to throw that out. I'm inviting you to find balance, so you can contribute in ways that are healthy and sustainable.

I'm not writing for the bootstrappers. They're not the ones reading this. They've never seen themselves as selfish. They pride themselves on being survivors, achievers. No, this book is for *us*: the community-minded women. The ones who worry that taking care of ourselves means betraying the people we love. The ones who are exhausted from holding everything together but still would never want to see it all fall apart.

We are not selfish.

We are the backbone of families, neighborhoods, movements. We love deeply. We give generously. But we cannot pour from an empty vessel, and we cannot keep sacrificing without intention or limit.

The Right Kind of Selfishness

Western mental health frameworks cannot be applied blindly. They must be critiqued and contextualized. And many of us in the field are doing that work already. If you want to dive deeper, *Decolonizing Therapy* by Dr. Jennifer Mullan is a powerful place to start.

But here is what matters now, the selfishness this book espouses is a reclamation of the word. I'm talking about a selfishness that is rooted in *love*. Love for community and love for self.
Finding the way to pour into both will sustain your healthiest self. And why does a healthy individual matter? Your health will elevate the community you love. You will pass down generational wisdom. Generational ease. And how do we do that? We don't pass the healing work to the next generation like a hot potato. We do the work now. We share a blueprint for health. The title may lead some to believe I am encouraging you to reject community. I am in fact encouraging you to be the reason community flourishes.

Let's get practical.

Step 1: Know your values.
Write a list of your core values. *You* must be in the top five.

Step 2: Track your time.
Write out how you spent the last day or week. Where does your time, energy, and money go?

Step 3: Ask, "Is it working?"
Does how you spend your resources align with your values?

Step 4: Adjust.
Move things around. Make small shifts. Make hard decisions.

Step 5: Stay in community.
Ask yourself: Am I staying connected? Am I accidentally isolating? Are my relationships reciprocal? Am I welcoming healthy people as I release the ones who harm?

Step 6: Keep checking.
Balance is active, not fixed. And remember: discomfort isn't always a sign of danger. Sometimes it's a teacher.

Sacrifice will always be part of building and maintaining community. But it should be
intentional, consensual, and *sustainable*. Not automatic. Not expected. Not blind.

Before you give, ask:
Am I participating in a communal exchange, or an individualistic one?
Is this contribution nourishing or depleting?
Am I giving from free will, or obligation?

Let your selfishness be your compass.
Let your community benefit from your healing.

~Reflection Page~

Conclusion

Let's Heal Ourselves with Selfishness

We have to live differently or we will die in the same old ways.
— *Alice Walker*

Protect your spirit, because you are in the place where spirits get eaten.
— *John Trudell*

Why did they call you selfish? Was it a mirror being held up for your betterment, or was it a trap, meant to keep you ensnared in servitude and exhaustion?

We've explored how community and connection will require sacrifice. But now, we are intentional. We have identified our priorities and made a commitment to save enough for self. We have chosen to be selfish.

You are unpacking what you were taught, looking at the rules you were handed but did not help create. Now, you get to decide what stays and what goes. You recognize that burnout and martyrdom do not define womanhood. You do.

The world has created a nightmare and disguised it as a fairytale. We've been told, over and over, that love is pain, that romance thrives in imbalance, that proof of a woman's love is staying long enough to change someone. But none of that serves healthy relationships. It only serves the machine: patriarchy, heterosexism, and the myth that our worth lies in our ability to endure.

Those machines are grinding us down, our bodies, our spirits, and our relationships. So now, we must be selfish. We will ask questions, define what feels nourishing, and pursue that.

The price is clear. We now understand that the silence we keep and the burdens we carry are not simply about keeping the peace. The status quo is making us sick. Being selfish is about physical survival. Our mothers taught us that stress will kill us, and the science is catching up to what the mothers knew.

In choosing to be selfish enough to survive, we also choose to communicate more clearly, to set boundaries that protect our energy, to prioritize health and replenishment. We are learning to listen to our bodies, early and often, before the consequences become dire.

It's okay if you don't know how to love yourself yet. This book is an invitation, not a test. We began a conversation to explore what it could look and feel like to truly care for yourself, without shame, without guilt, without apology. You deserve care. You deserve to live. It takes time to get to know yourself, and that time is well spent. I encourage you to skip the shame of not knowing and commit to trying. Try new ways of showing up for yourself until it feels right.

Be what they said you were, be selfish. You will never win everyone over. Some people are only comfortable with your depletion. Someone who is okay with your suffering for the sake of an institution will never see things your way. And that's okay. They don't have to.

We are saving our own lives.

We are building new systems. Improving on the idea of community, one that includes healthier people and more balanced relationships. Don't wait for someone else to see you clearly. They may never say, "I see you. You are the backbone of this. You've made so many sacrifices." The great thing is their clarity is not required for our progress.

The higher goal is for you to see yourself. See yourself as good. As worthy. As a full participant in the community you love so deeply. The only person who needs to see you right now is you.

Be selfish for her. Take a stand. Reclaim your resources. Make sure she is safe and healthy. Once she is cared for, reflect. Learn how to protect her. Then return to the world, knowing that you will be called selfish for surviving, but also knowing that your return, as a healthier version of yourself, will benefit even your critics.

What the old guard doesn't understand, or refuses to admit, is that it's not "us or them." Choosing yourself doesn't mean rejecting your family. Caring for yourself doesn't mean abandoning responsibility. We aren't striving for self-centeredness. That's the other extreme, and like most extremes, it's not sustainable.

This is about balance. The resources we keep for ourselves and the boundaries we build are not about shutting people out, but about building something solid and lasting. A structure that supports not only us, but everyone we care about.

There is a win-win. It may be less straightforward than "us or them," and it certainly requires more work. But a balanced self who mindfully contributes to a healthy community is a vision worth the effort.

Journal Prompts for Reflection

- What does it mean to you *today* to "be selfish"? How has that definition changed since you started this book?

- In what ways can you begin saving your own life right now? What needs to shift?

- What old beliefs are you ready to let go of, and what new truths will you carry forward?

- What would it look like to see yourself clearly and act in alignment with what you see?

- If you believed you were worthy of care, how would you live differently?

The woman who's always been the rock, the bridge, the balm You deserve to be held, too.
You deserve to be full.
Let them call it selfish. But you and I both know the truth: You are not

selfish. You are saving your own life.

~*Reflection Pages*~

www.ingramcontent.com/pod-product-compliance
Lightning Source LLC
Chambersburg PA
CBHW072136070526
44585CB00016B/1702